What Doesn't Kill You, Makes You Stronger:

One Woman's Insight
On The Ups And Downs
Of Living With Cancer

—

And Beating It!

Kate Henwood

DEDICATION

For Ollie……the one I do it all for, my reason to get up every day..

CONTENTS

ACKNOWLEGEMENTS

My story began its life as a emailed blog, for my friends, when I was diagnosed with cancer in 2015. Previous experience of the cancer journey taught me how exhausting it is, physically and emotionally, to explain, over and over again, what's going on, what the test results were, what the consultant said.....and it's boring!! (I became a cancer widow in June 2012 when my husband Bruce died after 14 months of oesophogeal cancer that spread to his liver, abdomen and brain. He was just 50, our son Ollie was just 10 when his daddy died). I blogged when Bruce was ill and I knew that I needed to do it for my journey too. It was cathartic to write and get everything that was playing out in my head onto paper…

The blog grew and evolved into a Facebook page, Kate Can Do This, where I posted the blog and where my friends could get involved. It meant that I could try and keep my cancer separate from my other Facebook "life"…..

Cancer is what I have, it's not who I am.

My mission, through my blog, was to raise awareness of what it's really like to live the cancer journey, because having and dealing with cancer is not always like the medics and the professionals tell it – usually because they haven't been on the rough end of it.

It's also my mission to show people that a cancer diagnosis doesn't have to stop you from living – it may shorten your life, but it DOES NOT have to stop you from HAVING a life.

My goal is to make the cancer journey easier – easier to face, easier to understand, easier to deal with…..if I can make a difference for just one person, then I've succeeded.

There are so many people that I need to say thank you to.....

Richard Simcock, my oncologist; Riccardo Bonami / Charles Zammit – consultant surgeons responsible for my surgery; Lynette Awdry – my wonderful friend and mentor in all things cancer-related; the Chemo Team – Lou, Katrin and Annie; Jo Hull, my Acupuncture therapist; the fabulous medical team at The Montefiore Hospital in Hove, who have looked after me every time I walk through the door.

My Mum, Chris and my amazing son, Ollie – just for being there and giving the best hugs ever;

Gay, Bev, Kay, Jane, Penny, Penny, Amanda ,Jane, Dawn, Lesley – my brilliant friends and "minders" who have been with me every single step of the way and without whom I could not have coped with this journey;

Paul & Zena, Ollie's godparents, who have been there for Ollie, throughout my treatment;

Sue, for welcoming Ollie into her home and making him one of the family, whenever I needed a break; to Maria and Gino for their amazing hospitality and fab Italian coffee; to Luke and Grace for being the most amazing, supportive friends to Ollie;

Linzi, my therapist, who has taught me so much about "being" rather than "doing" and has worked with me to kick my cancer and get me to optimum health, both during my treatment and into the future.

March Marvels – a wonderful group of ladies - my online buddies, all of whom were diagnosed with breast cancer at the same time as me.

And to all my friends, both local and online, who have written the most amazing words, messages and encouragement, been there and offered help and chocolate when required.

1. LET'S START AT THE VERY BEGINNING....

In early January 2015, I found a lump in my left boob.

Getting it checked out, the GP I saw believed it was probably hormonal. An appointment was booked for 3 weeks later to recheck. Needless to say, it was still there. A hospital referral was duly booked for 10th February for investigations.

This is my story.

10th February 2015

Ok. So today's appointment confirmed what I already suspected......

Having had a mammogram, ultrasound and 3 biopsies, consensus of opinion is that the lump in my boob is cancerous. There may also be some lymph gland involvement. This will all be confirmed next Friday (20th) along with the CT scan I'm having on Thursday. From there, we work out a treatment plan, which will either be chemo then surgery or vice versa.

For now everything goes on as planned, within reason.

Ollie knows everything and is being amazing. If he talks to you, he knows as much as you do and always will.

I think that's all for now - except to say that this is just a process - we deal with it and move on. I have a trip to Florida booked for Dec 2015 and I will be on that plane.

Love you all and thank you for being there!

2. TODAY IS THE FIRST DAY
OF THE REST OF YOUR LIFE....

16th February 2015

So today I saw Mr. Bonomi, the lovely Riccardo, and got the results of last week's biopsies and CT scan.

As I suspected, the biopsies show that the cells removed both in the breast and in the lymph glands are grade 3 cancerous cells, which means that they are fast growing. The CT scan also shows an abnormality on the liver and lower spine - further MRI scans next week will show whether these are cancerous or whether they are just abnormal cells, along with the bone scan that's booked for Monday.

The consensus from my medical team is that we will start the process with chemotherapy under consultant oncologist, Dr Richard Simcock, at The Montefiore Hospital in Hove, where I used to work. This could be as early as the end of next week.

After chemo, we move to surgery, probably a double mastectomy, followed by radiotherapy and then reconstruction when my body has had time to recover.

So that's the technical detail - what about the people involved in all of this?

Ollie, as when Bruce was ill, knows all the information - he's a smart boy, who NEEDS to know what's going on and we don't have secrets. What he needs is normality, not questions (ask me, not him please) - he's 12 and been through all this already. He needs to know that a cancer journey CAN have a positive outcome. He will need support, fun, laughter, friends and at times, a taxi service!

And me, I need to back off the majority of things I do and look after me. The quickest way I'm going to recover from this is to be entirely selfish. I will need people to play taxi for me and to help me - being fiercely independent, that's going to be very hard.

I need friends around me who support the way I'm walking this journey and I'm fortunate to have a some very special and close friends who I can rely on 100% - you know who you are and I love every one of you.

This blog will be updated whenever I've had an appointment - from experience, it saves me having to explain to people when we meet - we can talk about way more interesting stuff than what my blood count is!

Most importantly I need you to be "normal" around me.....please don't stop inviting me to things and ask me about stuff....let me make the decisions over what I can and can't do. I can't guarantee that I'll be able to turn up to stuff, I might only stay for an hour and I may cancel at the last minute.

I know for the majority of you this is a huge shock and you might not know what to say and I get that...I've had a month of getting my head around the fact that something wasn't right. You don't need to say anything at all.

God has a plan.....I just have to go with it!
Please keep Ollie and me in your thoughts and prayers (if praying is your thing).

Love and hugs to you all xxxx

3. AND BREATHE....

19th February 2015

This evening I went to meet with my oncologist, Dr Richard Simcock, to talk about my treatment plan. Although there's no "new" information about what the scans and biopsies showed, now we have more detail. The tumour in the breast is in excess of 9.5 cm, about the size of a tangerine and the two in the armpit are about 5cm each. That's kind of shocked me.

The other concern are the two anomalies in the liver and spine, which could mean that the cancer has already spread; these need further investigations and that means MRI scans on Tuesday. If this is the case then we're playing a whole different ball game.

Results from the MRI scans will be available next Thursday when I see Dr Simcock in clinic again, when my treatment regime will be decided.

What we do know is that chemo is the way forward and it

will be a 3 week regime (chemo once every 3 weeks via an IV drip), starting Thursday 6th March.

So now we have to wait and pray........hard......

This is the difficult part........I don't do "waiting".

The last few weeks have taught me to sit.....to sit with the things that hurt, that don't fit into MY plan, to sit with things that I don't want to deal with.

Right now I'm having to sit with a potential situation that I never ever wanted to face, that I haven't asked for.....

I can do nothing about it.....I have to hand this up to God and wait...

I have to be "in the now" because that's all there ever really is........

.........and breathe..........

Love and hugs to you all xxxx

4. TESTS, SCANS AND BRILLIANT FRIENDS....

24th February 2015

So yesterday I spent all day at the hospital - spinal MRI scan in the morning and a liver MRI scan in the afternoon, interspersed with a 5 mile hike round Brighton and Hove with Kay & Jane, to use up the 4 hours that I wasn't allowed to eat for, before the second scan! I'd never had an MRI scan before and didn't really relish the thought of the confined noisy metal tunnel - needless to say it was ok.....something else to tick off the list and something that will no doubt be repeated on this journey.

The latter end of the day saw a visit to the chemo unit to discuss, plan and prep me for the chemo regime that starts next week - things have changed slightly in that chemo will be a Tuesday, not a Thursday. We still don't know what drug regime - this will be decided tomorrow once we have the full reports from the various scans, tests and analysis.

We also sorted out the insertion of my Port-a-Cath - the permanent cannula that the chemo will go through - it means my veins stand a chance of surviving chemo and it can also be used for blood tests, fluids and anything else that needs to go in or out of a vein. This will happen on Friday afternoon under general anaesthetic, ready for chemo on Tuesday.

I suppose because the chemo regime is something that I lived through with Bruce, this visit didn't really bother me. Don't get me wrong - I'm not looking forward to it, but it is only a process - a means to an end - it has to be done. The staff on the unit are lovely - I worked with Lou, the chemo unit sister, when I was at Spire, and in turn, she was at the Nuffield when Bruce was there - it's kind of gone full circle - I'm in very safe hands. It helps that we have the same warped sense of humour - my laughter therapy mentality will be actively encouraged! Maria, my breast care nurse, is lovely too - she's my "go to" person at the hospital for all the worries relating to treatment etc. And that means that although the lovely Lynette is at the hospital & I'll see her whenever I'm there, she's there as my friend and not as a part of the medical team - I couldn't do this without her or any of my brilliant friends, who are already eternally in my debt - you know who you are and I love you all! xxxx

Last night saw a great evening, catching up for a curry with Bev & Penny - I was starving! We talked and laughed about everything - normal stuff - it was just what I needed and will need right the way through treatment. It's all too easy to lose sight of the little things that make a big difference - I don't want my life, and especially Ollie's, to be dominated by this journey - it has to, to a large degree, but there are still so many other things that are going on, that I don't want to miss out on, I just have to adapt and find ways to make things work!

Today is a relatively normal day - not one hospital appointment and I get to network with some of my Mumpreneur friends in Arundel this morning - woo hoo! I have a jobs list to the moon and back to do before chemo on Tuesday - most of it won't happen but we can try!

I think that's all for now - your messages and posts are brilliant - keep them coming.

Love and hugs to you all xxxx

26th February 2015

Ok........thanks for all the posts and messages this morning - going into Facebook radio silence now until I've got my results....really need to focus and just be in the moment.....

Keep the prayers and positive vibes coming......today is a massive day.

I promise I WILL post later on and let you all know where we're at.....it may take a while to form any words that actually make sense.

Love you all and thanks for being there xxxxxx

5. RESULTS….AND WHAT NOW?

26th February 2015

So………today was the big day…..results…..The last 24 hours have been…….challenging…..

We knew that the cancer was in the breast tissue and in the lymph glands in the armpit. The best case scenario was that this was contained and isolated in the breast tissue.

The CT scan picked up anomalies in the liver and spine and this is what the MRI's were for - to identify if these anomalies were a threat or not.

The absolutely brilliant news is that the liver anomaly is completely harmless - it's like a liver birthmark.

The not so great news is that the spine anomalies are bone cancer - in 3 places - lower spine and breast bone.

BUT the good news is that it is treatable but it's not

curable....it can be treated and managed long term, by way of a 4-weekly injection that makes the bone cells inhospitable to the cancer cells. It is highly likely that I will need more chemo later on, but that's way down the line, and possibly radio therapy to the affected bone areas.

So the treatment plan is as we discussed last week - chemo intravenously every 3 weeks from this coming Tuesday for 6 cycles (18 weeks), then it will be a bi-lateral mastectomy and then radio therapy, along with the 4 weekly bone cancer-related injections. So by the beginning of December 2015, the breast cancer should be dealt with and gone.....the bone cancer will be being controlled and closely monitored.

So tomorrow I go in to hospital for the port to be fitted and then it's all systems go for chemo on Tuesday.

Yes, we all prayed for a better result, but hey, let's face it, it could be soooooo much worse.

Thank you so much for all your lovely messages and posts, presents and cards and most of all for all the offers of help and lifts and everything - I love them all and they carry me through the dark times. Please keep them coming, they make a huge difference!

Love and hugs to you all xxxx

6. AND SHE'S BACK....

28th February 2015

Apologies for the lack of blog yesterday - honestly, it would have made no sense.....anaesthetic has a lot to answer for!

Yesterday was a day that saw me back at the hospital - I've been there more this week than I've been at home!

The port-a-cath (it's purple! How great is that!), enabling me to preserve my veins while I'm having chemo, is in and working; about the size of a Quality Street triangle, and buried in my shoulder, just below my collar bone, this is a little valve that the medics can use to give drugs and take blood - basically anything that needs to go in or out of a vein can go through here!

Mr Salman, the lovely man that did my op, was so conscious of where to place this. He made sure that, as a driver, it wouldn't get in the way of my seatbelt and that as a lady (allegedly!) the scar wouldn't show outside the neckline of tops and dresses - 10/10 from the stylist in me!

I opted to have a general anaesthetic (could have had a local but I'm a bit wimpy), and forgot that me and GA's have an odd relationship. Coming out of it was highly emotional - when your body is out of your control, things just "happen" - the tears flowed for what seemed like forever.

Tears are a good thing, learning to let go of all the emotion that's built up and will build up on this journey. It wasn't the first time and it won't be the last. Sandy, my nurse in Recovery, was fantastic, as were all the staff that I met yesterday, holding my hand and wiping my tears, giving me the space to cry for as long as I needed.

By 8pm, having been fed and watered, dressing changed, painkillers taken and instructions on aftercare given, I was on my way home - huge thanks to Jane and Kay for my chauffeur service yesterday!

Getting home felt good; greeted by a huge hug from Ollie and a cup of tea for both Jane and I. I can't tell you how proud I am of Ollie - at 12, he shouldn't be going through this, or stepping up and being the most marvellous support I could ever ask for.

So having caught up with the most important call I had to make yesterday, to my wonderful Mum (who was diagnosed with breast cancer herself 14 years ago when I was pregnant with Ollie), without whose love and support this would be so much harder, and all the messages and Facebook posts, my bed felt heavenly and thanks to the right drug combination, I slept! First time in 4 nights - not brilliant   sleep   but   chunks   of   healing   sleep.

Healing comes in many forms - the hospital and drug treatment form a major part and I'm so grateful that all of my medical team not only support, but actively encourage, the use of holistic healing at every stage of treatment. They even having the services an acupuncturist onsite, who I'll be seeing onsite, as acupuncture is proven to relieve some of the side effects of chemo.

Because of this support for holistic healing, all the fantastic work that I've been doing with my wonderful therapist, Linzi, can carry on and carry me through this journey, with her support and guidance. Another wonderful person in my life - it's so about having the right people around you.....

Today will be brought to you by Tramadol and tea and rubbish TV - I can't drive til Monday really, with the drugs and anaesthetic, so I'm not really going anywhere - although I quite fancy a walk round the block later if anyone is free.....I feel I should take someone with me.

Thank you for all the offers of help.....when we really get into treatment, I'll be asking for help left, right and centre!

Love and hugs to you all xxxx

7. CHEMO'S BEEN DELAYED....

2nd March 2015

Quick update......tomorrow should have been the first chemo session but it's been delayed. Although I'm psyched for it, the reasons for the delay are good. The HER2 receptor results that we've been waiting for are back and positive. (HER2 is a protein that determines how the cancer cells grow and divide and there are some really effective targeted treatments that work really well for HER2+ cancers). This wasn't what the medical team was expecting and is great news as the results of chemo on this receptor are really positive. Because it wasn't expected, the chemo that I need has to be ordered and won't be here til Thursday.

It is also a different regime and will need some heart tests before I can have it. If these can't be fitted in before Thursday, we may need to do part of the regime this week and the rest next week. I still need to go to the hospital tomorrow as there's new stuff to sort out and also my first session of acupuncture. So not quite the week I was expecting but at least it's only a bit of a delay and not a week!!!!

I'll update again when I know more.

Love and hugs to you all xxxx

3rd March 2015

Going to look at wigs tomorrow......not sure whether to go with something similar to how my hair is now or to do something completely different......your suggestions, folks?

8. CHEMO 1 – AND WE'RE OFF….

5th March 2015

Well that's Chemo 1 complete – 1 down, 5 to go………

This week has seen good news with the HER2 receptor result and the start of acupuncture, as well as apprehension about how chemo will go. Although I walked this journey with Bruce 2.5 years ago, walking it for yourself is very different.

Normal life carries on – on Tuesday, Ollie and I were choosing his GCSE options at school – he has made some great choices and if he gets those subjects in the final selection, he'll be a very happy boy. I'm so so impressed with the maturity that he's showing, with school, my situation and life in general – a definite "proud mummy" moment.

On Wednesday, Gay and I had great fun visiting Gary at Creations Hair Salon in Chichester, to choose my wig. I've said that as soon as my hair starts to come out, it's coming off. I got offered the cold cap treatment to preserve my hair but I know that my hair would still thin and it's fine enough already. It's a great opportunity to have a play with what I might like to have after it grows back too.

We chose various ones in a variety of lengths.....the wigs will be here on Thursday night so I can make my choices! Watch this space for the photos!

Because the HER2 results didn't come back till Monday and were unexpected, my chemo prescription (Docetaxel) changed and I couldn't have it on Tuesday. It also meant that I needed a heart scan before I could have 2 of the drugs (Herceptin and Pertuzumab) – these two drugs block the HER2 protein which is the instructor chemical that tells the cancer cells to grow.

Richard, my oncologist, decided that he wanted me to have these drugs now, rather than wait.....he didn't feel I was at undue risk and so the 6 hour observation period after I had them was crucial. As it happens, I had a phone call mid-morning to say that they could do the heart scan later that afternoon anyway, so that has saved me a trip down there next week and got the final tests, for this bit, completed.

So having got to the hospital at 9, I got home at 7; thanks to Jaz and Sean for feeding Ollie!

My port worked brilliantly, after an initial hiccup when it didn't want to play. At least my veins are being preserved from having a cannula inserted every time!
It was a long day, and they also gave a loading dose of everything the first time, to give it a kick start. That means

that subsequent sessions will take less time, which is good. I was so lucky that I had my good friend Jane with me all day, and Lesley popped in too, so I had company and loads of laughs!

The staff on the unit are lovely – I knew Lou, the ward sister, from our previous journey – we have a similar sense of humour (!) and Elaine was my dedicated nurse for the day and she was lovely too. Nothing is too much trouble and we were furnished with drinks whenever we wanted them and lovely food at lunch time. This could be a grim process, but attitude and the way you are treated make so much difference.

Along with steroids, anti-sickness drugs and Piriton, to stop me reacting to the other drugs, that's my drug cocktail complete. I have an injection to administer at 5pm on Friday evening, then 3 days of steroids etc., then nothing more till my next chemo session on 24th March.

Who knows what will happen in that time……this is where I step into the unknown on my journey…..a time to be "in the moment" and do what feels right at that time. With regular acupuncture sessions booked and working holistically with Linzi, I know that I'm doing everything I can to lessen the negative effects of this chemo regime, and promoting the best environment for the chemo to do its job in dealing with the cancer cells and shrinking "IndieGo," (IndieGo is what I named my tumours….I vowed to love them because if I loved them they would go away and being angry with them would be negative and not conducive to healing. I visualised them and I got the colour Indigo (hence "Indie"). The "Go" was part of "go away" and "God" – "go away" was the action that I needed and "God" will be a major contributor to their going away – hence

"IndieGo"). There are events in my diary for the next 3 weeks…..all of them are subject to feeling ok and being able to get there – there may well be last minute change of plans or cancellations….it's part of the process, the need to be flexible and "go with the flow". I also have to be very aware of other people's health…..my immunity will take a blow, even though I'm boosting it with my eating regime, so if folks have colds or bugs, I need to know as that could determine whether I go to stuff. I'd rather know and miss something, than pick something up and then my treatment get delayed or compromised because I'm not well enough. So if we're supposed to be meeting up and you aren't well or think you've got a cold etc., please can you let me know – then I can decide and make a judgement call on whether I can take the risk or postpone for another day – that would be great, thanks!

So I think that's all for now…..the journey to recovery has begun; it may not be a straight road but the destination is in sight….. (42 weeks or 289 days until Ollie and I fly to Disneyworld - YAY!)

Thanks for all your support, messages, prayers and offers of help for me and Ollie – they are all greatly appreciated and will be invaluable in the next weeks and months.
Love, prayers and hugs to you all xxxxx

9. CHEMO 1 – DAY 4….

8th March 2015

Chemo Day 4 and I'm doing ok......... Thursday was a long day and I crashed out at about 8.30pm and slept till about 2am.......Friday started early.....

I think I'm just going to have to rearrange my day round my body clock rather than trying to make my body clock change - it knows what it needs and I just have to listen to it.

Friday was kind of a normal day.....popped into town to get my nails done - I had to take my gels off before I had the port put in and have felt naked ever since. Chemo can really affect your nails, like it does with hair, and having gels back on will help to keep their strength for a while, at least till the existing nails grow out. I couldn't decide what colour to have so I went for the rainbow effect!

Friday afternoon was spent at work, planning world domination and recording the next two style videos and just being "normal" - I just love my job - we ALWAYS have a laugh and Friday was no different.

Ollie had a friend over for a sleepover - it's great - they entertain themselves and it really helps Ollie cope with all that's going on. I can't begin to tell you how proud I am of him and how he's coping.....

By 7.30pm I was exhausted, but in a good way..... the post chemo steroids are great for keeping you going but it means that, although I was exhausted, my body wouldn't sleep till about 11 pm. Then I only slept for 2 hours and awake for 3 hours, and then dozed till early Saturday morning.....oh, and in the wee small hours, it appears I've registered for this year's Race For Life.......if you want to be one of "Kate's Angels" - it's 5 days after my final chemo session (hopefully!) - we will be walking, not running, and will be in a lot of pink, and angel wings!

Despite the erratic sleep, Saturday morning felt good and the boys decided that swimming and lunch in town was the order of the day.

Having dropped them off, a bit of retail therapy and a catch up with friends over a cuppa filled a bit of time before Mum's Taxi was summoned to pick up the boys. I think I lost an hour during the afternoon.......the body decided I was tired, but not before some brilliant advertising opportunities and negotiations for work.....

Ollie's social diary meant a birthday sleepover at a friend's - and a night alone for me.......yes, I was in bed by 8pm! Amazingly I was asleep by 9.15 and didn't know anything till 6 this morning - RESULT!!!!

Just as an aside.....last night I thought, because Ollie was out, I'd treat myself to a takeaway.....I thought I fancied a burger......when I went to eat it, it was awful.....there was nothing wrong with it, but I've really got into my smoothies and "proper" food again and I just couldn't eat it......I'm afraid it went in the bin and out came the green smoothie. Lesson learnt.......

So Sunday morning looks good, the sun is out and I'm feeling ok. Ollie needs collecting at 9 and I might just get to church this morning......there's a lot to say thank you for, right now.

Love, prayers and hugs to you all xxxxx

12th March 2015

Chemo is a funny thing....it affects things you'd never imagine......yesterday I was moaning (sorry Linzi, observing with attitude and acceptance!) about my sore nose and acne skin. So today I decide that natural remedy was best for the aforementioned spots......within 30 seconds of applying a minuscule amount of tea tree cream to my chin, all I can taste is tea tree!! Eugh!!

Oh and just observing that I now appear to have a cold......now it's a sore red runny nose......still the Echinacea throat spray tastes better than the tea tree! On the plus side, it's 8.15pm and I haven't fallen asleep today. I must be feeling better!

10. CHEMO 1 – 2 WEEKS ON….

19th *March 2015*

So we're now Chemo 1 and 14 days – the next dose is coming on Tuesday. The past week I've felt human again…..most of the time. I think the hardest part is trying to balance the seesaw of "I feel great, let's get loads done" and "I've done too much, now I feel rubbish" – it's SOOOOO hard! By Cycle 6 I'll have it cracked!

I've been through a raft of side effects – the constantly runny nose, the flu-like symptoms, feeling sick, no appetite, sleeping, not sleeping, utter exhaustion, being awake at stupid times, sore hands and feet, craving Marmite(!!) – in some ways it's very like the early days of being pregnant.

One of the odd ones is that I can't eat anything that is hot in temperature or hot (as in spice / flavour). If I do, it makes my mouth and face burn - and makes my skin go all dry and flaky, like windburn! So it's a rather restricted diet at the moment as I can't have any dairy (because it's not recommended for breast cancer) – I can often be found chomping on a chunk of cucumber, rather than chocolate etc.......visualisation is really great when what you really want is CHOCOLATE!!!!!

The medical team at The Montefiore are great and I have their full support when it comes to using complementary therapies. I've always been into homeopathy and having a holistic take on life. This has really come into its own now and I'm open to all sorts of ideas and "alternatives".

What I've experienced from chemo is all chemical side effects – using natural remedies, rather than more commercial pharmaceutical drugs, makes logical sense to me, and I'm blessed with knowing some awesome therapists who are making this process so much easier.

I'm using homeopathy to counter the chemo effects, along with weekly acupuncture, that the hospital advocates.

Because food is a real issue for me, I'm having to really listen to my body and what it really needs.....this week it's been food that cools.....the chemo makes the inside of me hot, so to cool it, I need cool food – makes logical sense really!

I've been working with a wonderful lady called Linzi since April last year, using massage and yoga and now, everything that we've been working on together (and it IS a partnership) – breathing, attitude, presence, being, letting go – has all fallen into place; without working with Linzi, I would never have been able to "sit" with my ankle injury and accept it, or to "just be" with my cancer diagnosis. Eternally indebted, Linzi – thank you.

Meeting Linzi in January 2014 wasn't by chance ....you all know my theory that everything happens for a reason and that we have people in our lives for a purpose......this was one of THOSE meetings.

Last week I went to Creations in Chichester to see about wigs.....there's an 80% chance that I'll lose my hair so I'm getting in ahead of the game and getting my wig(s) now! It's a great opportunity to have a play with hairstyles – the lovely Gary, Gay & I spent a great hour, looking at styles and generally having a laugh. Tomorrow I get to choose what I'm going to have, out of the 8 I ordered in. It's very tempting to go for something very wacky......... because I can get away with it! Watch this space....I suppose you could call it "Wig Watch"!

Yesterday I was up in London, networking with 200 fantastic female entrepreneurs at The White Company and The Mumpreneurs Networking Club. Chemo makes my immunity to germs very low– yesterday was not the best thing for me to do and yes, I'm exhausted today, but it keeps things "normal" – I got to see loads of friends and I'm so glad I went.
With cancer, life goes on if you let it and it doesn't have to take control. There are times when it comes first and other times when it really has to learn its place!!!!

You guys have been SOOOOOO supportive – it's great. Not one day goes passed without a text, message, Facebook post etc. from someone, reminding me to stay strong etc......keep them coming, it's great.

Don't forget ladies, it's not too late to register for the Race For Life. I know 1000's of women around the country are doing Race For Life – all the money goes in one pot......please DON'T feel you have to sponsor us – if you sponsor someone, then you are doing your bit for Cancer Research – every penny takes us closer to finding a cure for this mutated cell that devastates lives....... (I'll get off my soapbox now ;-))

And Ollie, what can I say......I am truly blessed with a son who deserves so much praise.....he is amazing.......my rock and my reason for getting up every day. Please keep him in your thoughts too.

Please do share my blog on your timeline if you feel you can.....it's not for me, its purpose is to make others aware of what this journey is like, first-hand. It's designed to take the stigma and scare factor out of cancer – to make it less scary. Don't get me wrong, it IS scary but it doesn't have to be that unmentionable "thing".......if this blog helps one other person on this journey, then I will have achieved my goal.......

Enough from me – I'll be back after chemo on Tuesday.

Love and prayers to you all xxxx

20th March 2015

I'm moulting.........I was beginning to wonder if I'd be lucky and keep my hair....clearly not. No. 1 all over tomorrow then......
Anyone want to come with me?

21st March 2015

Well that's the hair sorted.....thank you Kay for coming with me and thanks to Sharmaine at SOTAS for doing the deed - this has to be the shortest we've gone! Beanies, scarves, hats and wigs all the way now!

Fantastic night last night in the company of Dawn's Vintage Do and Starlets Burlesque at The Regis Centre......first time in public with the minimalist hair - took me hours!

Thought I'd be able to cope with a night out but it completely wiped me out for today - need to learn to slow down......

11. CHEMO 2 – 2 DOWN, 4 TO GO….

24ᵗʰ March 2015

So that's Chemo 2 under my belt….the usual drugs plus one more – we've now added the Denosumab which is the 4 weekly antibody injection for my bone cancer. Basically it's to strengthen the bones and prevent fractures.

Mum came with me today, which was nice – being that she lives in Devon it was great that she could meet my medical team and at least have faces to put to names when I'm telling her who said/ suggested what. For me, her support is invaluable – she was going through this process herself when I gave birth to Ollie 13 years ago, so she totally gets where I am and what I'm going through. She was trialling Docataxel 13 years ago, thanks to her, I get to have it too, with the knowledge that it works.

I'm keeping a photo record of my cancer journey to run alongside the blog – yesterday Lesley from Infinity Photographic (http://infinityphotographic.co.uk/) took some lovely photos and I'll find it really useful to look back and see how far I've come and remember that there are loads of good days too – especially when I'm having a bit of a wobble…..if you've got photos that you take of me, I'd love to see them and put them in here….it keeps things "normal" for me!! If you can email them to me, that would be lovely!

I collected my first wig on Friday - ironically my hair started coming out on Friday evening so by mid-day on Saturday, I had dealt with that! It's so like my old hair and remarkably comfortable….You won't see it out and about for a while – I'm trying to get used to the "no hair" look as I'll be ringing the changes with my headwear at every twist and turn – the bald look, the beanies, hats, wig….I'll be keeping you on your toes!

So in cycle 2 I'm hoping / trying to get a bit more balance in how I feel – that means me doing less, listening to my body more, and planning less each day….that's the tough bit…..''No'' has to feature more, as does asking for help.

I'm looking forward to Easter and the run up to it – Lent and this time of reflection is really cleansing and with Easter being a time of "new beginnings", I really want to use it as a starting point for how things work for me moving forward….

So I think that's it for now……

Love and prayers xxxxx

12. CHEMO 2 – THE UPS AND DOWNS OF CHEMO….

3rd April 2015

Well, let's just say that the past few days have been interesting………

Chemo 2 went ok and the first days after were ok too; I didn't do TOO much and was mindful that I'd just had chemo…..after that, it all went downhill. By the end of Sunday I was in A&E at Worthing, feeling absolutely dire. All through Sunday I couldn't stay awake for more than 10 minutes and felt totally spaced out…..it was really scary.

I can't praise Worthing A&E highly enough……mention "chemo patient" and you're fast-tracked and top priority….because chemo kills your immune system, the risk of infection is sky high and infection will breed at a phenomenal rate. I'd been there less than 20 minutes and I was hooked up to 2 lots of IV antibiotics (don't get me started on that one) and had bloods taken and fast tracked to check for infection. If I had an infection, I would be staying in – no discussion.....Two hours, a chest x-ray, bloods and antibiotics later and I'm given the all clear to go home, except that my port wasn't cooperating......

A trip to the Montefiore on Monday sorted my port (which was fine, if used properly!) and also gave the opportunity for a long heart to heart with Lou, my fabulous Chemo Unit Sister.

When you travel this journey, everything is very practical. It's all appointments and drugs and regimes and blood tests......it's very easy to get dragged in to the whole thing and push aside the very personal side of the journey.....it's so much easier not to think about YOU as the patient and to just get your head down and get on with it......this week I've had to face some very personal fears.

I know I'll have to do this many times on this journey - I'm under no illusions. I'm also blessed with some wonderful friends who are holding my hand and walking with me.......this was one bit of the journey that I HAD to face on my own; having my friends on hand to support me while I did this was so important – not to judge or comment but just to BE there......

Part of the crisis on Sunday was sheer exhaustion.....not sleeping more than 3 hours a night is a killer and combined with chemo and all the side effects really does take it out of you. My sleep regime needs a reset and so that's being addressed too.

Yet again I'm having to revisit my diary...making sure that there are only essential things in it at the moment......going out for coffee and lunch count as essentials though!

And so hopefully the next few days will be a little calmer and productive and "normal".....

Have a wonderful and restful Easter......I'm hoping for dairy-free chocolate!!!!

13. CHEMO 3 ....

So that's Chemo 3 under my belt – in theory, there's only 3 more to go, assuming we don't have to move a session or have more chemo after the planned 6. It's always a possibility and I have to be realistic that this might happen.
I have an appointment with my Consultant on Thursday, so it'll be interesting to see what he says and thinks. I'm keen to know when I will be rescanned and find out what the chemo is doing. My gut feeling is that IndieGo is shrinking – call it optimism but my gut feeling has been right up until now.

So tonight, I'm feeling good. No chemo fog, no nausea, no falling asleep. For me, I do much better when I carry on as normal – whatever that is. So this cycle I'm going to try and psyche the cancer cells out, show them who's boss and carry on with normal stuff, but not too much of it......let's see what that does.

Cycle 2 wasn't great and it taught me loads – like you never know how today is going to be.....if I can't do something today, I can try again tomorrow and that I'm allowed to take time out to just chill and heal. I'm learning to listen to my body and give it what it needs. It's hard but it is great training for how I want my life to be when I'm better.

Yesterday I was presented with a beautiful hand knitted "Blanket of Love and Laughter" – masterminded by Kay and Jane, it's hand knitted squares, knitted by friends and strangers who have heard my story or seen my blog, making up a beautiful patchwork snuggly blanket that is perfect for those times when I need to cosy up on the sofa and rest.

It came to chemo with me today and it is soooooo warm. Thank you so much if you've been involved, I absolutely love it – I understand that there are enough squares for a second blanket – feeling very loved and humbled.......

So it's a short blog today – more after my consultant appointment on Thursday.

Thank you all for being so helpful and supportive – you all make my journey so much easier.

Love and prayers xxxx

16ᵗʰ April 2015

Just a very quick update......

I had an appointment with my consultant, Richard, this morning to review how I'm coping with chemo and the way forward. With 3 lots of chemo under my belt, I was keen to see how HE thought things were going.

Having established that, despite one trip to A&E during cycle 2, chemo so far has been largely uneventful. He asked how I thought things were and I said that I definitely felt that IndieGo had got smaller. A quick grope, sorry examination, brought a big grin to his face......IndieGo has indeed got smaller......not just a little bit, but in his professional opinion, by at least 50%......as have the tumours in the lymph nodes.

This is fantastic news and could change the game plan as he feels that by the time we have completed 6 cycles of chemo, there may be nothing to remove surgically!!!

Because the tumours have reduced so quickly, essentially after 2 cycles of chemo, Richard has suggested that we have a clip fitted to the breast tumour as a marker so that we can track it – bit like a micro-chip that you have for dogs and cats! This means that we can locate what, if anything, is left of the tumour when we eventually do the next scan. This will happen on Monday evening.

I think I've confused my consultant. My body isn't doing what he is expecting and I don't think he really knows HOW it is doing it!

Gut instinct says that attitude, positivity, love, friendship, good food, holistic treatments, prayers and laughter are making this happen.......please keep it going....it's working!!!!

So all in all, a really good day......

Love and prayers to you all xxxx

19th April 2015

Ok so today even water tastes revolting.......at least lime cordial is ok....for now!

5th May 2015

No chemo until tomorrow because of the Bank Holiday (one of my drugs has a very short shelf life and has to be administered within 24 hours of delivery....no deliveries on a BH!)

It'll be the same with the next one as that's after a BH too! But the good news is I need a haircut! My fuzzy hair needs shaving again as it's quite weak and if I cut it, the new growth will be stronger when it comes through. So it's back to the baldie look this afternoon!

14. CHEMO 4 – PAST THE HALFWAY POINT....

6th May 2015

So today was chemo 4 - blood tests were all good and I've been able to drop the Piriton so I'm not so dozy this afternoon. Chemo brain kicked in quite quickly - that moment when you know exactly what you want to say but the words just won't make it out of your mouth!

Cycle 3 was fairly uneventful, hence the lack of blog.....let's hope cycle 4 is as uneventful.....having said that, there's a few things in the diary, all of which I can cancel / postpone/ excuse myself from if I need to.....and my trusty Angels are very good at pointing out when I need to do that, especially as I will push myself a bit too hard at times.....to them I am eternally grateful.

Having said that I've just taken the dog for a 3k blow along a very windy seafront - it's still blowing a gale out there.....I've found that if I can give the toxic gunk they pump me full of on chemo days a helping hand to get out of my system, I do much better. The steroids I have just before and after chemo really muck up my sleep - this "walk" might just help tonight - fingers crossed please. Cookie should sleep this evening and not terrorise the poor cat!

It's windy weather like we have at the moment that makes you eternally grateful for eyelashes and nasal hair.....my eyes and nose streamed every step of the way - I wasn't crying - honest! Oh and I got bored with the hair growth that made its way through so I've had it all shaved off again!

And last Friday at The GlitterBall in aid of BabyBuddy, the long wig got its first proper outing and fooled everyone - no-one knew it was a wig so thanks to Gary at Creations for his excellent choice of wig and to Amanda for styling it so brilliantly for the occasion!

So that's it really - if you don't hear anything much, it's cos everything is going well and fairly normal. Fingers crossed that that is the case.

Oh and it's only 6 weeks till the Race for Life....I have 25+ people in my team for the walk, who have raised over

£1000 - how brilliant are they! It doesn't matter who you sponsor but please sponsor someone that's taking part, anywhere in the country....all the money goes to finding a cure for cancers..... any donations, from pennies to pounds WILL make a huge difference......

One final thing...if you're on Twitter, could you go and follow my page....I'd really like to get my blog out there....not for me, but to make this whole journey less scary for other people....."The C Word" BBC on Sunday did a fabulous job.....let's keep its momentum going......

Love and prayers to you all xxxx

19th May 2015

Acupuncture time with the lovely Jo from Essential Acupuncture - and then my bone strengthening injection.....it's all needles this morning!
Then back to work and an exciting day at the Style Studio, making new videos for the VIP style club and planning some amazing training

24th May 2015

We're nearly at Chemo 5....the side effects of the chemo are getting a tad frustrating......partially losing my eyelashes and being very light sensitive means my eyes water constantly so now we have watery eyes and a drippy nose.... I'm gradually losing the feeling in my fingertips - it's temporary - and for some reason, the flesh beneath my nail beds are all bruised. Try putting on socks or doing up buttons when you can't feel you finger tips and the nails are hurting...it's challenging....

But in comparison with some of my other "cancer friends", what I'm experiencing is minor...I'm still up and about, busy, able and being highly annoying.

Consultant appointment is on Tuesday night and chemo on Wednesday.....watch this space for the next thrilling instalment!

15. CHEMO 5 – HOT OFF THE PRESS....

26ᵗʰ May 2015

Today should be chemo 5 but it's not – it's been postponed.

I saw my consultant, Richard, last night – a routine visit to see how things are, symptoms, side effects etc.

I told him how rubbish cycle 4 had been – all my side effects have been worse and new ones have emerged, the nausea, even more rubbish sleep and the peripheral neuropathy in my hands and feet. I now have bruises under my nails and it makes typing etc. difficult – using a chip and pin machine hurts both fingers and bank balance and using a touch screen really needs a stylus now – I'm getting quite quick! It looks like I will lose the nails but fingers crossed, they'll grow back without too much damage to the nail beds.

His reaction was that cycle 4, 5 and 6 will be tough because my body is accumulating the chemo now, which is normal, and having to fight harder as well as being weakened by the general effects of the chemo. The up side is that my blood count is brilliant so the little soldiers in my blood are doing a fantastic job.

So I now have to feed a small army <u>and</u> a growing 13 year old!

But the reason for delaying chemo isn't because of any of this…..the obligatory examination (I'm sure this must be one of the perks of the job!!) left him with a big grin.

Subject to confirmation with a scan, it appears that all three tumours, including IndieGo, have GONE…..

Richard said when I saw him last time that this was a possibility….I didn't really believe that they would.

My scan is booked for the 7th July, to see the full extent of the 6 chemo cycles on the breast tumours and the bone areas that are affected.
From there, he will take all the results to his panel of experts where they discuss their complex cases – I have to be different! – and we can then formulate an action plan for the rest of my treatment and what is the best way forward long term, because we are looking at long term…..treatment of some description is a permanent feature, albeit in a less invasive way than chemo for now.

With all this in mind, chemo 5, which was due today, and chemo 6, will be reduced doses – in order to still hit the bony areas but to reduce the side effects, primarily the peripheral neuropathy.
The danger with giving the full dosage of the chemo is that

the peripheral neuropathy CAN become permanent and we want to avoid that at all costs.....at the moment it's reversible, and we want to keep it that way. High dose Omega 3 has been shown in the Cleopatra study to be highly effective in reducing the neuropathy so that's another thing I'll be taking.

So the delay to Chemo 5 is probably only until Thursday as the pharmacy need to reorder my drugs as they are measured dosage bags.

This will also mean that my final chemo will move 2 days, bringing it only 3 days before Race for Life – the upside is I'll still have steroids in my system and that should make the 5k walk a bit easier!!

Talking of Race for Life, Kate's Angels have raised over £1200 so far – we are now a 30+ strong team and have been chosen by Cancer Research UK to promote the race in the Worthing Herald and The Argus (hopefully). I couldn't do any of this without YOU, any of you.

Your prayers, thoughts, messages, texts, pictures and, in some cases, verbal abuse (I love it) and keeping it normal, (like I asked you to) are what makes this happen. So keep it coming – the next 6 weeks are going to be rough, but this cancer is on its way out, so let's kick it hard.

So it's chemo tomorrow hopefully......and maybe a small glass of something to celebrate, tonight.

Love you all xxxxx

1st June 2015

Sorry there hasn't been a blog after chemo 5. There wasn't anything to say!! All went well and no real side effects....or perhaps I've just ignored them.....
The fingers and toes are being a bit of a pain - constant pins and needles and I keep dropping things.....
One cycle to go.......it's like walking through a tunnel towards brilliant sunlight.....you can see the end but you're not quite there yet.....

4th June 2015

This is going to sound pathetic and shallow.....

I coped with losing my hair, feeling sick, everything tasting awful, tablets, injections, and the reality of a permanent lifetime cancer diagnosis and being uninsurable.

I've always had beautiful nails, they are my signature.....peripheral neuropathy and 5 doses of Docetaxel have decimated my nails.

I'm likely to lose at least 4 of them. Totally gutted.

I talk with my hands. I can't get a wig for my nails!! I guess I'll be wearing gloves a lot then....☐#chemosucks☐☐

6th June 2015

My lovely friend Claire sent me this article today (http://umberdove.com/blog/2015/6/4/warrior-blooded). It's all about how you face your cancer, how you treat it emotionally and psychologically.......at the beginning of chemo I resolved to love IndieGo, my tumour....to love her and send her on her way......and fingers crossed, she has gone on her way.......

Anger doesn't help when you're dealing with cancer...it just zaps more of the little energy that chemo leaves you with. And learning to love and care for your body is key....self-love, self-forgiveness, self-care......it's not selfish, it's absolutely necessary!

16. CHEMO 5 + 14....

Apologies in advance....this is a bit of a rant and a whinge.

Chemo 5 saw a reduced dose of Docetaxel (the chemo bit), because of the negative side effect of the peripheral neuropathy in my fingers and toes. The neuropathy gets worse with each cycle and it did the same this time. I flagged this up to the hospital early on so we wait and see if they reduce it further for the final cycle. Basically I can't feel the tips of two fingers on both hands and have permanent pins and needles in the others. Imagine freezing cold hands that are warming up...it's like that. My toes are similar - not as bad but it means I tend to lean back on my heels to get my balance.

I was lucky that I managed to preserve my finger and toenails up until now....chemo has caught up with them and they now resemble the nails of a 50-a-day smoker - they are revolting. Add to that the fact that the nail bed is dying underneath them.....2 nails are clearly infected as well as a toenail...I won't go into detail....but I may need them removed.....

The deterioration of my nails has rocked me more than the loss of my hair...it sounds shallow and vain, but I can't hide my hands while I have revolting nails or no nails....6 - 12 months of the constant reminder of what I've gone through.

Today I had my 3 month cardiac check - the Herceptin that I have, and will continue to have forever, can cause heart damage so these 3 month checkups are vital. All was good so that was a relief.

I spiked a temperature last night - the fluey symptoms that I usually get post chemo around day 4/5. I think it was just that I'd over done it yesterday and it WAS cold.....that rang alarm bells at the hospital today, so more blood tests were done and flagged up to the consultant, along with the deteriorating sensation in my fingers

The net result is that my final chemo, that should have been next Thursday (18th) has been deferred to the 25th, to see if the fingers recover a bit before we hit them again. When you do this journey you kind of hang a lot of weight on key dates. This has been a real target to aim for....now the flipping goal post has been moved. Gutted doesn't begin to describe how I feel. I understand why...it's just like someone's said "ah well, another week isn't that long". Trust me it is!!

The other gutting factor is the fact that where I should have been relatively symptom free for my birthday and weekend away, I'm now going to be at the stage where everything tastes awful......this Cancer thing sucks!!

On the plus side, I've been really lucky with my side effects, I've not had an infection or been hospitalised like a lot of my fellow fighters. So I shouldn't moan. But sometimes you just need to get it out on paper.....

Fingers crossed it doesn't get postponed another week - I really don't want chemo on my birthday!!

Catch you all soon xxxx

19th June 2015

Got a phone call from my consultant's secretary today....he wants to see me on Tuesday about my peripheral neuropathy, which is getting worse.....

I think chemo 6 may be on the line....And so I wait.....

23rd June 2015

Well that's the end of my chemo...oncologist says my neuropathy outweighs any further good the chemo could do and is very pleased with what the chemo has done.

He's moving my scan forward to next week and will see me with the results on 7th July and will schedule surgery for mid/end July.

Thanks for all your support....now we wait for the scan and results.

17. CHEMO 5 + 27....

24th June 2015

A lot can happen in 2 weeks!
Since my last post I've had 2 lots of antibiotics (for the gunky fingers and toes) and a dose of Herceptin and Pertuzumab, that made my peripheral neuropathy worse.

Conversations with the Chemo Unit and the consultant led to alarm bells going off about the neuropathy in my fingers and consequently I had a consultant appointment last night.

The shortened version of the story is that I won't be having my final chemo dose tomorrow - if I did have it, the chances are that my neuropathy would become permanent. In view of the amazing effect that the chemo (and all the other stuff I've been doing!) has had on the tumours, we felt that giving a final reduced dose of Docetaxel would not be a good idea.
So that's me done with chemo!

This means that we are able to bring forward the full body scan AND the results. My scan will be tomorrow and the consultant will take the result to the multi-disciplinary team meeting next Thursday and I'll get the results and the game plan on 7th July.

The plan is that I will have surgery for a double mastectomy sometime mid / late July and so I'll be recovering / taking it easy(!) for most of August. Radiotherapy will probably follow, either for any remaining traces of the breast tumours and/or for the bone cancer. The full body scan isn't expecting to show any change to the bone cancer - bone takes ages to show changes and so we will bone scan periodically in time. What we're hoping is that the bones haven't deteriorated.

In all of this I have one main short term goal....to be back to full health ready for our Florida adventures in December. Ollie really needs me to be at my best for this and I owe him that, at least!

After a good night's sleep last night, I realised today how much strain the whole chemo process has put on me. Today, I feel like I've been given my life back.

This is by no means the end of the journey - in some ways it's just the beginning. I have some amazing people that have been beside me on this journey, who have believed 100% that Kate Can Do This, even when I wasn't sure that Kate could.

Surgery is going to be challenging, not least because I'm going to have 2-3 weeks when I'm very limited in what I can do and being reliant on other people to do things for me. I'm going to have to ask for help.....

Laughter therapy and humour have played a huge part in my journey so far, and over lunch today we were talking about the fact that chemo has helped me on my weight loss plan for 2015.

As only close friends can, we got talking about how much weight I'll lose when I have my boobs off.....and so very soon you'll see my next charity fundraiser page go live.....it's your chance to have a guess at what my boobs weigh and raise some pennies for a cancer charity.....not sure yet which one. There will be a prize for the person closest with their guess....and yes there'll be a "booby" prize too. Watch this space!!

Oh, and a huge thank you to my 40 Kate's Angels who walked the Race For Life on Sunday....we raised over £3000! How fantastic is that!

Anyway, that's it for now.....go and enjoy this fabulous weather and check back in soon :-) xxxxxx

18. KATE'S DOUBLE TROUBLE CHALLENGE….

26th June 2015

In February 2015 I was diagnosed with secondary breast cancer - that means I have cancer elsewhere as well as in my boob. For me, this is bone cancer, for which there is treatment but no cure.....yet.

Having just finished 5 cycles of chemotherapy, I am now facing surgery to remove both boobs. Although it's only one that was affected by cancer, I'm not taking any chances. Life is too short to risk my health again and if it's good enough for Angelina Jolie, then it's good enough for me!

Now having been blessed (!) with more than my fair share of boob, this will be a weight off my mind, both psychologically and physically.

Ever since my diagnosis, I've vowed to bring something positive from the whole journey, be it raising awareness, dispelling some of the taboos and fears surrounding cancer or just showing that you CAN still have a life when you have cancer.....it's not the end.....in some ways it's the start of something new and very beautiful.

I've also been blessed by the support of many friends, without whom this journey would be so much harder. Among them are a core group of exceptionally special people who have held my hand every step of the way, picked me up, dried my tears, made me laugh, spurred me on, kicked my butt and kept things real. They have my eternal gratitude, love and I cannot imagine life without them. You know who you are xxxxxxx

But back to the point.......
When I have surgery in July, the breast tissue that is removed will be weighed. I'm challenging you to "guess the weight of Kate's boobs". Like I say, I was blessed, so there's going to be a fair bit to come off.

So have a guess, pledge some pennies for Breast Cancer Now (I'm suggesting a minimum £1 per guess), and join me in making the cancer thing a bit of fun.

Breast Cancer Now (http://breastcancernow.org) is aiming to ensure that by 2050, every woman that develops breast cancer will survive.

One in eight women in the UK will face breast cancer in their lifetime. And every 45 minutes, another woman dies from the disease.
Let's change those statistics......

19. SCAN RESULTS….

7th July 2015

So today was the BIG day.......

Seeing the consultant tonight was primarily to get the CT scan results - to confirm what we had already anticipated the chemo had done.....and it's all good news.

The 3 breast tumours look to have gone completely and the bones are responding to the chemo - bones take ages to show any change and Richard had already said he would be delighted if they had stayed the same - the fact that they have improved is a huge plus!!.

So the next stage is surgery for a double mastectomy. It's a big operation, in more ways than one, but one that I'm mentally ready for (I think). I see the surgeon on Monday for a consultation and surgery is booked for Monday 20th July at The Montefiore, where I've had all my treatment so far. I'll be in very safe hands.

After that I'll be restricted in what I can do for a while and also won't be able to drive for a few weeks, so I'll be asking for help.......

I've sorted Ollie for the last few days of term and then he is at my Mum's for a week and not home till 2nd August so he's occupied, which is great!

After that, I see the consultant again on 28th July and we are looking at radiotherapy every day for 3 weeks, in Havant.....the dates aren't set yet but will be mid-August. I may or may not be driving by then so might be asking for chauffeurs!

So by mid-September, my treatment should be complete and I'll be getting into a routine for the regular treatment that will (hopefully) keep the cancer away and keep me going for a good few years. There are no certainties, but we're working on a long term plan rather than a short term one!!

As per my last blog, the "Double Trouble Challenge" is still on! When I have surgery in July, the breast tissue that is removed will be weighed. I'm challenging you to "guess the weight of Kate's boobs". Like I say, I was blessed, so there's going to be a fair bit to come off.

Breast Cancer Now (http://breastcancernow.org) is aiming to ensure that by 2050, every woman that develops breast cancer will survive. One in eight women in the UK will face breast cancer in their lifetime. And every 45 minutes, another woman dies from the disease.

Let's change those statistics......

Please keep those prayers and positive vibes coming.....the next few weeks are going to be challenging and scary. But with all of you beside me, I know it will be ok.

Love and hugs

12th July 2015

Over the last few months I've read a lot of stories, where ladies have had breast cancer, treatment, lumpectomy, the all clear (as clear as it ever can be) and then the cancer returns, typically in the same place.

I've been asked a number of times in the past days and weeks, WHY I'm opting for surgery when my chemo results have been so good. And especially for a double mastectomy. "It's a big operation, do you really need to go through that?" "The chemo has done its job, is it worth the risks?"

Being entirely selfish, I don't want to go through chemo again. I don't want Ollie to go through chemo again. I will still have to have 3 weekly preventative treatment for breast cancer and injections for my bone cancer, forever.

I want to be around to see Ollie through school and college, settled, married, to hold my grandchildren, to spoil them rotten....

Surgery increases my chances of being around to do this.
It's not a decision I've taken lightly. It might not be the way you'd deal with it but this is my journey, my choice, my life.

And it's what I need to do.

This week I need to mentally prepare for this next bit of the journey and work through my own fears and concerns. Please hold me in your thoughts and prayers.

Sending you love and light.

20. APPOINTMENTS, APPOINTMENTS, APPOINTMENTS....

16th July 2015

Well it's all getting very real now!

On Monday I met with my surgeon, Ricardo Bonami, to discuss the game plan for my surgery. Having gone through all the options with me, making sure that I was fully aware of the scale of operation that we are undertaking, he agreed all the issues that I'd raised with my consultant and explained the ins and outs of my operation. My original diagnosis was one of inflammatory breast cancer – because this affects the characteristics of the skin as well as the breast tissue, reconstruction isn't an option for at least 18 months following a mastectomy. I'll be talking to my medical team at that point to see if I am going to have reconstructive surgery or whether I'm going to stay a member of the flat club!

Because I'm having a double mastectomy, I have the honour of having 2 surgeons working on me, one on each side. Both are excellent surgeons and will do a fantastic job. I did just throw in that it wasn't a race to finish and that I was expecting fabulous needle skills from the pair of them! In these situations, a sense of humour is essential, otherwise I'd be in tears permanently.

I'll be in theatre for around 2 hours on Monday, all being well, and I'm last on the list, going down around 4.30pm. Please don't expect any sensible comments or conversations on Monday!! Anaesthetic has a weird effect on me - I'm likely to cry.....a lot!!

Post-surgery I'm likely to be in hospital for 3 - 5 days.....it all depends how things go....this is going to be the hard part for me - being patient.....

When I get home, I'm going to be calling on my fab friends for visits and company....and the occasional trip to the shops or out for coffee.....I won't be able to drive for a while......that's going to be really hard!!

Ollie is coping so well with all of this - his godmother, Penny, is coming to look after him for another couple of days and then he's off to Paul and Zena's in Chidham for a couple of days, before going to my Mum's with his friend Alfie.

Knowing that he's occupied and in safe hands means I don't have to worry about him while I'm in hospital. I'm eternally grateful to everyone that's doing the "Ollie" duties!! Please keep him in your thoughts - he needs your prayers too as he does worry about his Mum, even if he doesn't say so!

So that's it for now......now I need to psyche myself for Monday.

See you all on the other side......

Love you all xxxxx

21. THE BIG DAY AND BEYOND….

20th July 2015

Having dispatched Ollie to school, made arrangements and organised things and people with military precision, taken Cookie to kennels and cleaned the house to within an inch of its life, it was time to go. Thanks to Kay & Jane for driving and escorting me to The Montefiore Hospital, and duly checked in and taken to my room - it was big enough to host a party!

Having been marked up and prepped for theatre, at 5pm, having walked to theatre, I was at the point of no return. At no point did I ever feel that I wasn't making the right decision for me. Four hours later I was back in my room, slightly sick and woozy, boobless but basically ok.....ok enough to text my Mum and closest friends to tell them I was ok.

Monday night was a combination of pain relief, observations, TV, intermittent sleep and conversations with my lovely nurse, Emma.

21st July 2015

So after a night of little sleep (no change there then!) and a complete bed change due to a leaky dressing, I've managed to get rid of the oxygen mask, the drip and the cannula in the back of my hand. That leaves me with a drain on either side, that I have to remember to take with me when I go walkabout!!

I've seen Mr. Zammit, the consultant, this morning - he was responsible for my right side - and he's very pleased with how surgery went. He'll be back in the morning to check on the drains and change the dressings, so I might get to have a look at his handiwork.

So now I just have to rest.......and recover. Thank you all for your lovely messages, I caught up with them late last night - they made lovely reading xxxx

I feel remarkably good - little pain from the wounds (more from the two drains that had been inserted), I have been able to get up and about and start my physio to ensure that I have good movement in both arms.

PS - ironically I chose melon from the menu for supper last night.....I did have a little chuckle to myself!!

22nd July 2015

Just had a shower - feels so good! Already seen the consultant this morning....my right hand drain can come out and my dressings can be changed...I get the first look at their handiwork - I can't wait to see the new look! There's a degree of swelling / puffiness on the left side, which will go, and I need to do some work on my abs (what abs, you ask! I can see them now, and my toes!)

The consultants were both very pleased with the way the surgery went - the results from the pathology lab should be back by the time I see Dr Simcock on Tuesday. These will determine the next bit of treatment and how much radiotherapy I'll have.

All being well, the left hand drain can come out tomorrow afternoon or Friday morning, and then I can go home! Craving fresh air and a seafront walk. We are so close to the sea here but the windows are sealed......

So grateful to everyone that has and is visiting and to my amazing friends who have been with me every step of the way - couldn't do this without you xxx

26th July 2016

Thursday was a very lazy day - I was exhausted and dozed for most of it......the anaesthetic had worn off and reality was kicking in. Talking to Mr Zammit (Mr Right Hand Boob surgeon), we decided that I would be able to go home on Saturday, assuming my left hand drain had done its job. Being that I was coming home on my own and not having someone to look after me, this was the sensible option.

And Friday was probably the lowest day - bored, fed up and shattered, thank goodness for Wi-Fi and my closest friends, who did their level best to keep me going from a distance - to them I owe a huge thank you - I was a very grumpy girl on Friday.....they didn't deserve the responses they got that day......sorry, girls xxxxx

On Saturday, following an early morning consultant visit, the final drain came out and I could go home! I can't tell you how well I've been looked after at The Montefiore....the staff, at all levels, are amazing and made the whole experience, which was massive in terms of the physical trauma and the psychological impact, calm and seamless.

Huge thanks to Bev and George for coming over to take me home. Just being out in the fresh air felt amazing - 5 days in an air conditioned building does give you cabin fever - although I had escaped down to the Chemo Unit to have my port needle removed! I felt like a naughty school girl, out of bed after lights out! So now I'm home and resting, doing little bits here and there, with supervision from my lovely "minders".

As I was reminded this morning, "just because you CAN, doesn't mean you SHOULD" - words that I will try and stick to as I recover from surgery.

Tuesday sees me back to the hospital, twice.....one for my 3 weekly IV infusion and then in the evening to see the consultant and get my results. After that, it's more of the same......rest and recuperation. It doesn't stop me from planning world domination, holidays, work, fun days out and having visitors. Do give me a call / text etc. if you fancy popping in - I'd love to see you, but I do need to rest......

Right now I'm experiencing loads of new things - being able to wrap a bath towel round me and it fitting, catching my profile in the mirror and doing a double take, seeing my toes, finding that half my wardrobe is miles too big.....little things.

For those of you who took part in the Double Trouble Challenge (AKA Guess The Weight of Kate's Boobs), the final weigh in was 7.45lbs and the closest guess was by Lizzy Von Tromp, whose guess was 7.5lbs. As was pointed out, that was the same weight as a friend's baby when she was born....imagine carrying that round on your chest for 33 years.......Amazingly, we raised £260 for Breast Cancer Now - it's a brilliant result so THANK YOU to everyone who took part in the fun!

Thank you to all of you for your messages, texts, prayers and love - they really kept me going while I was in hospital.

Love and prayers to you all.....

29th July 2015

It was all going too well......

And so I've spent this morning back at the hospital....yesterday's IV drugs made me really cold - chilled to the bone cold. Took me four hours to warm up. Felt better later but then it all kicked off in the wee small hours with a sky high temperature, shakes and shivers.

Waiting for blood results to come back and another course of antibiotics is highly likely - either oral or IV.

So lucky that my resident chauffeur, Kay, was free today to drive me and keep me company......

Watch this space......

22. PATIENCE….AND RESULTS….

9th August 2015

2 weeks in and things are slowly beginning to get back to normal.

My right hand side is healing nicely (after needing industrial strength antibiotics to clear up a wound infection) and I have very good mobility in that arm and shoulder.

The left hand side, where lymph nodes were removed, is taking longer and is still quite swollen. I had to have more fluid drained off last week but it's now healing slowly (Mrs Impatient is sure it should be healing quicker!!). It will be really nice to come off the painkillers soon - there's only so much a body can take and mine needs to detox from all the chemicals it's been fed!!

I saw Dr Simcock this morning to check over my wounds and healing - he's pleased with how things are going and both surgeons are pleased too. He also had the histology results from the surgery - my boobs have been under the microscope - literally!!

Samples were analyzed from the breast tissue and lymph nodes and the results are showing a complete pathological response. In layman's terms, this means that my aggressive chemo regime, prayer, clean eating, holistic therapy and positive mental attitude have kicked cancer's butt and.........

I NO LONGER HAVE BREAST CANCER!!!!!!!!!!!!!!!!!!!!

A truly amazing response to treatment - the kind of response that you dream of but don't dare to hope for........

We're not out of the woods yet......the breast may be cancer free but there is still cancer in my bones - that's not going to go away, but we CAN get that into remission - this will be through radiotherapy, beginning on 8th September - 15 sessions, Monday to Friday. The plan is to irradiate the bones in my lower spine but also to blast the chest wall and lymph nodes in my neck......it's going a bit OTT but it gives me the best possible chance of the breast cancer NOT coming back.......

Now I have to concentrate on recovery.....my body has been through a very tough regime of chemotherapy and 2 major operations......it needs to be nurtured and looked after, both before radiotherapy and after. It will be a good 6 months after radiotherapy before I'll be back to full strength - so I'll still be after favours and help here and there.

I have so many thank you's to say; there are too many to

say individual thank you's but you know who you are - I couldn't have done this without you......you've all been so supportive since my diagnosis....it makes a huge difference.

For now, I'm going to sign off and chill, enjoy the school holidays and look after me.

For now there's one hospital appointment every 3 weeks and a 4 weekly injection and a planning appointment for my radiotherapy......

For now, life can start to become "normal" again (whatever "normal" is!).......and long may it stay that way.

Love and prayers to you all.....

23. NEW TERM, NEW ROUTINE, NEW CHAPTER??

8th September 2015

So being that I haven't written a blog for a month, no news is good news. And as I'm sat connected to my drip, I thought I'd catch you all up.

Everything is healing well and life is starting to return to some sense of normality - Ollie is back to school, work is busy and active breast cancer treatment is nearing its conclusion. I start radiotherapy next Monday, daily for 3 weeks, in Havant, interspersed with my 3 weekly IV, acupuncture and consultant visits - it's going to be a busy 3 weeks but that's how I roll!

Radiotherapy is a whole new experience for me - the other bits of this journey I walked with Bruce; I kind of knew what to expect....this is new but I'm not worrying - there's no point, it achieves nothing!

Once radiotherapy and its side effects are over, I'm off to Fort Lauderdale on a business trip for a week - part work, part chill time. Ollie and I have a week away at half term, in a friend's caravan at Selsey and then it's only a few short weeks until we jet off to Florida.....and we can't wait!

Aside from that, I'm about to enter what I guess you can call a new chapter. Whilst my cancer diagnosis is never going to go away, I still have to factor treatment into my calendar - once every 3 weeks, I have the pleasure of seeing the amazing team at The Montefiore for my IV that will (fingers crossed!) keep my cancer at bay. This element is permanent - quite a sobering thought when others that you have been walking the journey with are now celebrating being cancer free. Don't get me wrong, I'm not bothered by it.....it's just how it is and sometimes it smacks as being unfair.....let's face it - it could be a whole lot worse.

With all of this in mind, it's time to say a huge thank you to you all for holding me and Ollie in your thoughts and prayers over the last 7 months....the power of prayer and positivity I'm certain has had a direct result on my recovery. Now I'm going to ask that if you've had me on a prayer list at your church, please could you consider taking me off. It's not that I don't want / need your prayers, but moving forward I'm not anticipating needing any more prayers than anyone else. I'd love to say thank you to your congregation personally, but that's just not possible, but if I could say thank you via your pew sheet or newsletter that would be great - please feel free to copy and paste the following paragraph, if you wish.......

"Following 7 months of chemotherapy, surgery and radiotherapy, I'd

love to say a huge thank you to everyone for your prayers, thoughts and messages during my treatment for breast cancer. The results have been amazing and the breast cancer has now gone...the bone cancer appears to be responding well and is being controlled by injections. I have been truly blessed with this response and give thanks to God for this amazing result and for everyone that has supported me on this journey.   Kate Henwood "

So now it's on with the show and really looking forward to starting this new chapter and experiencing whatever it may hold......

Love and prayers to you all.....

14ᵗʰ September 2015

So this is day 1 of 15. Day 1 of targeted radiotherapy. Day 1 of taking the train from Worthing to Havant. Day 1 of a 15 day countdown to the end of active cancer treatment.

From then on, my treatment will be regular and planned and preventative. Routine. Predictable.

8 months, a fantastic medical team, medical science, holistic therapy, prayer and a whole bucket load of positivity have taken me from facing a disease that would probably have killed me, to facing a bright, positive, healthy, happy, LONG future, a very different outlook on life and a whole bunch of wonderful friends, without whom I couldn't have walked this journey.

Who's ready for the next chunk of my journey??

17th September 2015

I was writing my journal this morning and talking about cancer being so much more than a diagnosis and also trying to put into words how cancer can make you feel.....this sums it up I think....

Taken from Harry Potter and the Prisoner of Azkaban: "Dementors are among the foulest creatures that walk this earth. They infest the darkest, filthiest places, they glory in decay and despair, they drain peace, hope, and happiness out of the air around them... Get too near a Dementor and every good feeling, every happy memory will be sucked out of you. If it can, the Dementor will feed on you long enough to reduce you to something like itself... soulless and evil. You will be left with nothing but the worst experiences of your life."

Cancer can do this.....but only if you let it. Treat it like a Dementor....ward it off with the happiest memories, your most cherished thoughts and experiences. And eat chocolate.....it keeps Dementors away.

18th September 2015

Radiotherapy week 1 of 3 complete.....for those of you that have never seen a scanner, this is what it's like. The breath hold technique that is needed to keep the lasers from damaging my heart requires this medieval instrument of torture - I didn't like this bit of scuba diving - I dislike this even more....

21st September 2015

Day 6: 10 sessions to go....think the side effects are starting to kick in. Tastes are still all over the place....metallic mouth.....and now my digestive system is being affected by the radiotherapy to my spine....definitely not feeling the love this morning.

22nd September 2015

Back at the meat handling plant. Pushed and pulled around to get the positioning right. I know it's crucial but please remember I have feelings and emotions. They seem to have been forgotten today. Very nearly lost it in the scanner today - images were being reviewed as I lay half naked on the table, not knowing what was going on, not being told anything until later on. Seriously folks - communicate!!

Seriously not sure how much more I can take. And please, no one tell me I've only got 8 more to go. I'm likely to lose it completely

24th September 2015

So 2 days after an awful radiotherapy session and a quiet word with one of the other staff, I had the most lovely session today, an apology and a full explanation of what they were concerned about. I saw the images that they compare daily, I found out what the staff do and see when I'm in the scanner and all is well again. Hugs all round and just 6 sessions to go....

Thank you to everyone who messaged, commented and showed me that it WILL all be ok xx

29th September 2015

12 radiotherapy sessions down, just 3 to go.....

24. THE END OF A CHAPTER....

3rd October 2015

So Friday saw my last radiotherapy session....a long three weeks, probably the hardest 3 weeks of the whole process.

Not physically but emotionally draining because there's no let-up.....it's in your face every day.....

But I did it.....with support from some amazing people, who stopped me from throwing in the towel half way through (I was that close) and some brilliant friends who rocked up and came to Havant with me - thank you, it really did make a difference.

Alongside the radiotherapy, I've been put back in contact with the Penny Brohn Cancer Centre which is an amazing centre that educates and works with those who have a cancer diagnosis, showing them how to LIVE with cancer, rather than allowing cancer to control their life.

(http://www.pennybrohn.org.uk/).

Those of you who walked this journey with Bruce may remember that we went to Bristol on a couple of occasions to learn more about how to live well with cancer. On the other side of the fence, I'm hoping to go back there in the new year, for me this time instead of as a carer and hoping that my very dear friend will come with me for support.

With the end of radiotherapy comes the end of active treatment. While many see this as a time to celebrate, it's actually quite daunting.

For the past 8 months, I've been engulfed in an endless round of appointments, scans, tests, drugs, treatment, advice, medical intervention and hospitals. You don't really have time to digest and process it all - it just happens TO you. And although everyone tells you that you have choices in your treatment, when your consultant, who you trust implicitly, suggests a course of action, you tend to go with it.....not without questioning it, obviously, if you're me, but your heart tends to lead you.

It's by no means the end of treatment though.....now we fall into a routine of treatment.

Now I'll have a bone scan in February, see my consultant every 6 weeks, and have a CT and cardiac scan every three months for the next 12 months. After that, if there is no evidence of any changes, then we can make those tests and appointments less often.

I'll also have 3 weekly IV of monoclonal antibodies to try and prevent the breast cancer cells reactivating, a 4 weekly injection to strengthen my bones.....for life or until they stop working.

My biggest challenge right now is to reconnect with my body and making it mine again. 8 months of tests, poking and prodding, every medic you see wanting, needing to examine you. You leave your dignity at the door when you are diagnosed, stripping off for a consultant becomes routine.

If you've ever watched "Les Miserables", it's reminiscent of the scene where Fantine prostitutes herself and takes herself off to a happier place. You go into autopilot every time because your body is no longer special. Cancer strips you of your dignity, your hair, your nails, your breasts.....everything that identifies you as a woman. And still you carry on.....because you have NO choice. None. It's not about being brave or strong or inspirational. It's about fighting to survive. Because you have to.

Essentially now, life gets back to "normal". I have to say I have no idea what "normal" will be.

It won't be the same as before, it can't be. It'll be slower, because living life at 100 miles an hour does me (and you!) no good. All I do know is that life is for living and that I have to put myself and Ollie first in what I do from this point forward.

So now we move from one chapter to the next. I don't think I can ever close the door on this chapter because there are still bits that need to be revisited and with cancer the door is never fully closed. But the next chapter is going to be exciting....very exciting!

From now, the blog will be less frequent, but I'll keep you posted!!

Love and prayers to you all......

9th November 2015

Some days are tougher than others......today seems to be one of them.

Nothing has happened, no tests, no results, no reason to be down. It just happens....

Tomorrow is my next IV - nothing to worry about. I just don't want to go and have it done. I guess it's just the fact I HAVE to do this, to help prevent my cancer coming back.

Days like today are the days when it's easier to put on the mask and be "strong" rather than to be brave and let the tears flow.

Tomorrow is another day when normal service will probably be resumed.

Let's hope so.......

2nd December 2015

So yesterday was a hospital day......my usual IV and then a CT scan......the first since chemo and radiotherapy finished.

People have asked if I'm worried....it's a tricky one.

I feel great, yes, and I'm getting back to doing what I did before. Probably doing too much and learning by my mistakes.

I'm learning to listen to my body and it's telling me that things are ok, good in fact.

But yes, I'm worried. Because I felt OK BEFORE I was diagnosed.

So until I see my consultant next Thursday I WILL be worried, quiet, possibly snappy ......for which I apologise now.

Or I might well act like everything's fine because sometimes that's easier than trying to explain exactly how I feel...

So it's fingers crossed all the way to next Thursday, with lots of coffee and cake along the way.

25. RESULTS DAY....

10th December 2015

It's a while since I've blogged.....and not a lot has happened. I'm still having IV preventative treatment every 3 weeks and an injection every 3 weeks - it's just a routine now. Tamoxifen drug treatment starts imminently because my breast cancer was hormone positive.

Like you, we are getting ready for Christmas and our holiday and trying to get work finished so that it truly is a holiday. Without wanting to preach, Christmas isn't about presents, it's about presence......this year, more than before, I've learnt who my friends are......my Christmas wish is that YOU spend time with those who are important to you, tell them you love them, don't assume they know.....

I had my regular CT scan last week, to check the full extent of chemo and radiotherapy.....I saw the consultant today and he had some good news. The chemo and radiotherapy have done what he hoped......bearing in mind that my bone cancer is incurable, treatable but not yet curable. We knew from the pathology results from the mastectomy that there was a complete pathological response i.e. successful treatment of the breast cancer.. The CT scan shows that the bones are responding to the preventative treatment and as of today.........

I AM OFFICIALLY IN

REMISSION!!!!!!!!!!!!!!

Happy bunny doesn't start to describe how I feel.........and huge thanks to everyone who has supported me in 2015....I really couldn't have done it without you.

So here's wishing you all an amazing and peaceful Christmas and a brilliant 2016.......

Love and prayers to you all.....

26. 2015 – OVER AND OUT....

30th December 2015

Posting this today as we'll be at sea tomorrow and out of internet range:

So 2015 draws to a close. What a year! Did I imagine this time last year that 2015 would be the way it's been? Never!

I was looking forward to the first part of my Styling course at LCF in London in early January and then a full on year, with Gay and I having big plans for Style Me Confident in its 10th year.

Did I imagine that falling off a kerb just 7 days into 2015 would radically change not only the next few weeks but the rest of the year and ultimately, my life.....um, NO!!!! But it did.

My cancer diagnosis came on Feb 10th – a date I will always remember – not because of what happened but because it was my Mum's 70th birthday. The day I had to tell her "Mum, I've got cancer". What a shit birthday present that was!

The plans I had for 2015 went on hold and a whole new timetable came into play. Many many times this year, when things have had to change, I've been reminded of one of Father George's phrases – "when WE plan, God laughs". He's so right! The path we travel is pre-set. But the way we travel it is not.

For me, 2015 has been a year of change, both physically and mentally.

Thanks to chemo I've lost 3.5 stone and my hair – my new hair is thicker, stronger and darker (The weight isn't coming back!). Thanks to surgery I've lost both boobs and the lymph nodes in my left arm, some movement and sensation, but even that is coming back, with patience and expert support.

I've lost the plans I had for 2015. I've lost control of my life. I've lost people from my life that I thought were my friends. You could say I've lost this year to cancer.

There are a lot of losses in those last sentences.

Have I gained anything from this year? Hell yeah! So much it's difficult to know where to start.

The twisted ankle in January was telling me to "slow down" – I was told that if I didn't, it would take me way longer to heal and get back up to speed. Did I listen? Well, kind of…..my cancer diagnosis forced me to slow down. I had little choice – my life revolved around hospital visits and treatment, although I did manage to negotiate those to my timetable most of the time. Fortunately my consultant has the patience of a saint and when he says NO, I do have to listen.

Having to slow down has made me re-evaluate how I do things and even IF I do things. And that's been hard.

I've had to ask for and accept help. That's been really hard, although I'm getting better at asking now!

Self-care is a word that's been around a lot this year and I've become very selfish, for which I offer no apology. I have to look after me in order to do the things that need to be done and the things I want to do. To be around as Mum AND Dad for Ollie, I HAVE to put myself first. That often means that if there are 2 things going on in a day, I have to choose which one I can do, not assume I can do both. And that's hard too.

Ollie – what can I say about Ollie? To lose one parent is devastating. To lose two is plain careless. All joking aside, this young man has been my daily reason for doing what I do, throughout treatment and beyond. I don't think he'll ever know how he's helped me through all of this but he has. And his friends have been there for him too and I'm eternally grateful to them.

I'm one very proud Mum – always have been and always will be. Ollie has the world at his feet and I'll move heaven and earth to help him become whatever he wants to be, because the secret in life is to do the things that you're passionate about, the things you'd do day after day, without pay, and still feel passionate about them.

I've gained some amazing friends and some of the amazing friends and family that I already had have stood by me, picked me up, held my hand, been to appointments with me, driven me everywhere, dried my tears, got me drunk, fed me cake, spoilt me rotten and nagged me relentlessly.....because they care.....and I love them for it. You know who you are......and you've made this year so much easier than it could have been.

"If I could turn back time......" - would I change this year? There's a question.....

I wouldn't wish cancer on anyone. I've been lucky – my breast cancer treatment has been successful and is, as much as it can ever be, a done deal. You can never say it's gone but I have had a complete pathological response. That's as good as it gets. The treatment for my bone cancer is working, it's under control and so long as I keep up with my treatment, that too is in remission. Until a cure is found, I will always have cancer. Yes it's life limiting, but just like everyone else I don't know when my time will be up. I just have to be a bit more careful with what I do and how I do it! If you read the medical statistics I might have 5 years. Me? I was always rubbish at statistics. I'm just working on life being long and full and fun. I've got way too much to do to be disappearing anytime soon!

But would I change 2015? Hell no!

I've learnt so much about me, about my friends, about life, about what's important and about what really doesn't matter a jot.

This year I have become stronger, feistier, and more

stubborn (if that's possible), but I've also become softer and more open. I've learnt to trust again and be vulnerable (and in turn, brave) and I hope, become a better person.

My blog has reached 1000s of people and I hope helped some of them, be they on this journey or walking with someone who's travelling this road. And I have developed an abject "dislike" of the word "inspirational" - I'm just me!!

So with 2015 on its way out and 2016 on its way in, I'm making no resolutions and no major plans – God has all the plans – I just need to TRUST and enjoy the ride. Oh, and enjoy every minute.

So here's to 2015 – thank you for every lesson that you have taught and everything that you've shown me.

And 2016, let's see what you have in store for me.

BRING IT ON!!!!!!!!

27. MOVING FORWARDS....

14th January 2016

Just been to see my surgeon for my 6 month check-up post-surgery and I'm pleased to report that he is delighted with my healing and range of movement.

He's disappointed that my scarring is not as pretty as he would like but I always scar badly.

He did say he could arrange something cosmetic if it bothered me but to be honest, my scars have healed nicely - let's not mess with them!!

I asked him about the amount of pain and tenderness I still have.....apparently it's the equivalent of being trampled by a herd of elephants....it will take time to go.....it could be 18 months before it fully settles down.....I have to be patient......I give it 6 months to stop hurting....

My other concern was the tightness in the arm pit......this is because of the incision to the muscle and tendon and the effect of the radiotherapy to the chest wall. It will improve with time and massage and stretching.......thank goodness I have my wonderful therapist in my corner.

My range of movement was a concern to me....I was worried that it wasn't that great. He said I shouldn't be able to do what I'm doing for at least 18 months.....there are times when I really wish I didn't set my own bar so high.....

The really good news is he doesn't want to see me for another 12 months....unless I want to see him.

So now I need to concentrate on recovery, keep pushing the boundaries and keeping the bone cancer at bay, in remission and in its box, where it belongs!!

Thanks for walking this journey with me....it felt like you were all at the appointment with me - boy was it crowded in there!!

28. LIFE IS A ROLLERCOASTER....

28th January 2016

As Ronan Keating says "Life is a rollercoaster, just gotta ride it......" and boy, do we ride the rollercoaster.

After an amazing trip to Florida and a once-in-a-lifetime (well maybe not) cruise over Christmas and the New Year, we hit January and 2016 with a bump. Having had some health issues over the New Year, my step-dad, Roy, went into hospital 10 days ago and will never come home....he was diagnosed with bladder cancer and scans show that it has spread to lymph nodes elsewhere. It's terminal, there is nothing they can do, except keep him comfortable. Roy came into my life when I was 5 – we're not amazingly close, but he's always been around, which is more than I can say for my biological father who is conspicuous by his absence.

So now I am trying to support my Mum, long distance

(they live in North Devon), as she comes to terms with, or tries to, the impending life trauma of the death of a husband / wife / partner. And let's face it, she's had cancer herself, lost a son-in-law to it, been through it with me, and now faces losing her husband to cancer – it really isn't fair!!

For me, it's reliving those days and weeks that you exist through, waiting for the inevitable – I call it "life in the bubble" – stuff is going on around you but you're detached from it….you're on autopilot. You're wanting the end to be quick and pain-free but feeling guilty for even wanting it……you make plans for "afterwards" and then worry what other people will think about the decisions you make. It's awful! So I'm sending huge hugs to Mum – it gets better, eventually……

Please hold us, as a family, in your thoughts and prayers at this time.

Tuesday was a hospital day and unusually my port (the magic button that all the drugs and bloods goes through) was being a pickle. At the 3rd attempt, it granted us access and everything was fine. Until Tuesday evening, when the whole of my right shoulder, neck and chest wall decided they wanted to join in. After a night of no sleep, pain and palpable pain in my neck, I phoned the hospital, went in, got it checked and a scan booked for today – to check if the port had moved / fractured / failed – and came home.

One of the skills that I've learnt this last year (and am still learning) is to quiet the "monkey chatter" in my head – that incessant voice / ego that butts in and asks awkward questions and makes you doubt everything. Working with Linzi, I'm learning to quieten the monkey, close the box in the left side of my head that it lives in, go into that empty box on the right hand side and just wallow in the nothingness that it holds…..to be……to really be present….really be "in the moment".

Last night I went through every "what if" scenario that exists……what if it's failed / needs replacing / hasn't failed / there's a tumour……my "monkey" went ballistic with all the possibilities – it was horrible and emotional and irrational…….and perfectly normal.

So today, when my scan showed that the port was perfectly alright (I'd seen the images!), not failing, moved or damaged, my monkey went into orbit! If the port was fine then the only explanation was a huge tumour in my neck; after all, that's how Bruce's secondary tumours started…….

Richard, my oncologist was in clinic today and, thank you Universe, had just finished with his last patient, as I came out of my scan. Within 5 minutes I was being examined, poked, prodded for anything untoward……his other specialty is head and neck cancers (I am so lucky to have him as my consultant!!). His verdict was that whatever is causing the pain in my neck, it's nothing to be worried about…..it will go as soon as it came, in his professional opinion. If he's not worried, then neither am I – I trust this man with my life – literally. He said, when you have a cancer diagnosis, your default setting with ANY lump, bump, pain etc. is to assume that "it's come back"......totally totally normal – horrible but normal. He's told me he'd rather check and scan me every time, rather than have a patient worrying needlessly or missing anything that needs to be dealt with. This man is worth his weight in gold.....and more. One "monkey" calmed (eventually) and a very emotional Kate, who managed to keep it altogether (until she got back to the car, and then the floodgates opened!!).

I'm so grateful to Linzi for showing me HOW to put my monkey in its place.....it's a skill that I will constantly be practicing and using......Linzi, you're a lifesaver!

So, for now, the rollercoaster of life keeps rolling – and I'm just gonna ride it! Who's coming with me??

Love and prayers to you all.....

Kate xxx

ABOUT THE AUTHOR

Hello, I'm Kate.

Kate the mother, Kate the widow, Kate the friend, Kate the business woman, Kate the taxi driver , Kate the victim. Poorly Kate, camera Kate, theatre Kate, the 'can I have a lift Kate?' & sometime 'sexy wig-wearing Kate'!

I'm Mum to Ollie, chief animal feeder & walker, in charge of all domestic arrangements and in my professional life - Administrative Director of 'Style Me Confident'. This is my story, well the bit from where I fell off a busy London pavement while taking on a spot of professional development. The bit from when I'd recovered from this slapstick accident, only to be told that I had cancer - big, fat, proper, life altering, ugly, miserable, cancerous cancer. And not just one variety, oh no – a most unreasonable range of cancers! I try not to do things by halves, as you can probably tell.

So here it is, my journey thus far, with cannulas & chemo, Disney & dearest friends and of course, my boy. And this is how I travelled.

Hello I'm Kate, and I firmly believe what doesn't kill you makes you stronger.

16005315R00065

Printed in Great Britain
by Amazon